YOUR KNOWLEDGE HAS VALUE

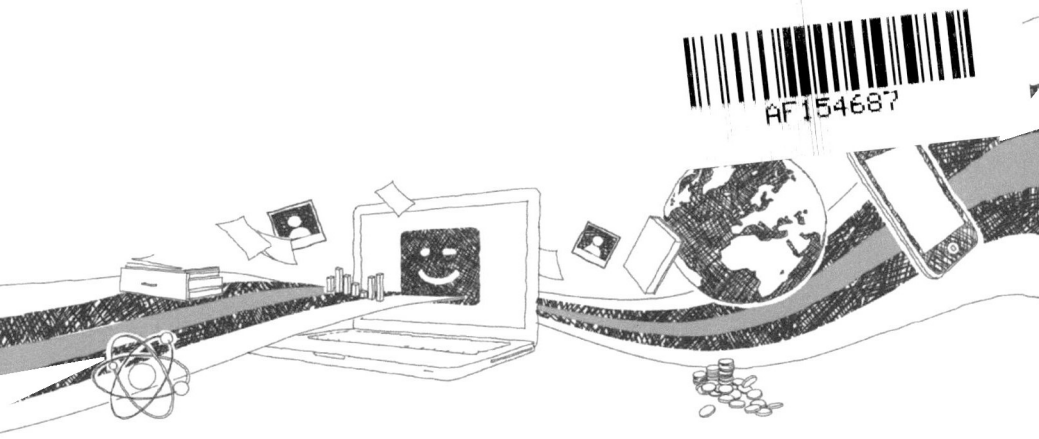

- We will publish your bachelor's and
  master's thesis, essays and papers

- Your own eBook and book -
  sold worldwide in all relevant shops

- Earn money with each sale

Upload your text at www.GRIN.com
and publish for free

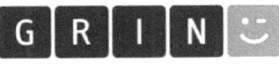

Bibliographic information published by the German National Library:

The German National Library lists this publication in the National Bibliography; detailed bibliographic data are available on the Internet at http://dnb.dnb.de .

Imprint:

Copyright © 2013 GRIN Verlag
Print and binding: Books on Demand GmbH, Norderstedt Germany
ISBN: 9783656531852

This book at GRIN:

https://www.grin.com/document/233347

Mukasa Aziz Hawards

Enviromental Impact Assessment: An Approach to Public Health Management

GRIN Verlag

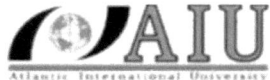

Name: **Mukasa Aziz**

Course Name: **Environmental Impact Assessment**

July 2013

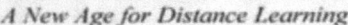
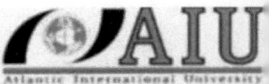
Table of Contents

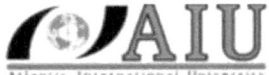
Course outcomes

Description

The course in environmental Impact assessment concentrates on identifying the major factors responsible for environmental stability and instability, ad methods in determining or estimating the extent of their effect. Therefore this course; prepares the ability for identifying, developing and implementing effective solutions to environmental challenges, especially in an international context.

Course objectives

The learning outcomes of this course study include knowledge and understanding of a range of environmental topics as well as intellectual, practical and transferable skills and competences, as detailed below;

* ❖ Acquire knowledge of current scientific theories, paradigms, concepts and principles of natural and human-induced environmental processes that are essential for formulating modern environmental policies.
* ❖ Gain understanding of existing political, economic, legal, international, and social implications of human interactions with the environment
* ❖ Understand environmental policy processes and principles of effective environmental governance as well as main factors of environmental politics.
* ❖ Learn how the private sector can handle environmental issues and mainstream the environment in business strategies.
* ❖ Understand the basic principles of environmental assessment, auditing and life cycle assessment.
* ❖ Understand the purpose, scope and limitation of key methods by which environmental and related information can be gathered, processed and interpreted
* ❖ Learn the key social factors that impact the environment.

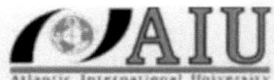
Literature Review

Our environment is a key defining factor that can be used to establish and to predict the health status, economic progress and downfall, social and economic development, human interactions and quality of regulation and policies operating in the given community or at the national level.

Though environments may vary from one to another in terms of health status, bio-diversity, pollution, and extent of exploitation by human activities, economic value but yet in even when these factors are present all environments share a fundamental feature which is their ability to support life and hence they provide reliance for man's natural existence.

Though science and technological advancements are changing the trends in environmental support and reliance to man's existence, yet all these inventions are always aimed at devising means of increasing and boosting the support of the environment towards man and for his wellbeing. Any threats and endangering of the human environment both to the biotic and abiotic components does not actually exert its effect on the environment itself but rather onto those that are supported by it. The concept or idea is that the environment only exists for our good and t no time or extent has the environment turned negatively impacting to man unless destabilized by man himself.

This idea therefore, is elaborative of the implications of man to the environment and not that of the environment because it is man who is supported first or in other words human existence emerges from the environment. Science has it well explained through the topic of ecology that for an efficient and reliable eco-system to exist, both man and the environment must exert a positive impact to each other to a particular extent. This is because the eco-system is made up of biotic interrelations namely; food webs, food chains, and energy flow cycles.

This study is a scope therefore, into these environmental dynamics and its relevance to health is vital not in mere theoretical approaches but more so in the general practice for every person but we are all stake holders when it comes to environmental; protection, dependency and reliance. Achieving a positive human environment that is supportive in all spheres of man's involvement and enjoyment there is need to analyse the state or status of the environmental exploitation and degradation and responsible use of it at an international scale.

This study presents research outcomes and revised approaches that can be applied in assessing the impacts of the environment to human health and existence and after this it outlines elaborately the various policies and strategies that have been and can be used to change the negative and threatening impacts of the environment onto man and his future existence.

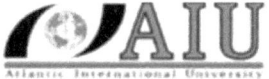
Chapter One

Introduction to Biodiversity and Eco-Systems

The human environment can also be regarded as the natural environment in which variety of biodiversity is found to interrelate and cause impact to each other. The biodiversity of the natural environment is regarded as the life consuming factors which also include both plants and animals. There has been a social neglect in the understanding of the components of biodiversity where man only concentrates on the plants and animals.

Biodiversity is treated as a contraction of the term "biological diversity" and according to Luc Hens biodiversity can be defined as the variability among living organisms from all sources including, inter alia, terrestrial, marine and other aquatic ecosystems and the ecological complexes of which they are part; this includes diversity within species, between species and of ecosystems" (CDB).

There are so many living organisms that are not necessarily plants or animals but falling into other categories of the living organisms. Consider the main kingdoms below in which all the living organisms are categorised;

1. Kingdom prokaryote; this kingdom is sometimes referred to as monera and it comprises of tinny unicellular micro-organism that lack an organized and enveloped nucleus. These organisms also lack a variety of membrane bound cell organelles.
   The common example of organism in this kingdom is the bacteria whose size ranges in diameter from $0.2\mu m$-$4\mu m$ with the length from $0.3\ \mu m$-$10\mu m$ and from this size it can only be seen with an aided eye while using magnifying lenses (Principles of Biology). The role origin of the bacterium is essential in the study of human science because it offers the basis for the evolution of man and the disease micro-organisms.
2. Kingdom Protista: this kingdom is mainly composed of protozoans and other simple multicellular. There distinctive feature is the organized envelope for the nuclear material such as the genetic composition for the organism. These organism play a vital role in the establishment of efficient food chains and food webs in the aquatic life and in other types of eco-systems. The common of these are the planktons, amoeba, paramecium, euglena, and zooplanktons. This kingdom also contains self-supporting organisms called algae that have pigments that trap sunlight which provide the solar energy used in the synthesis of their food e.g. the spirogyra (Concepts in Biology).
3. Kingdom fungi: this kingdom comprises of heterotrophic organisms that live as parasites or saprophytes. Most of them are multicellular but a few are unicellular.

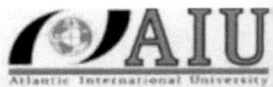
The bodies of the multicellular fungi consist of a branching system of threadlike filaments called hyphae. The common examples to man's routine environment are the rhizopus, mushrooms and the mucor. The fungi are common environment factors in medicine and nutrition hence they are of principle importance (Biology, Advanced topics 4th edition).

4. Kingdom plantae: this is a common group of organisms which are characterized by their ability to synthesize food with the help of the chlorophyll pigment.
   Plants are basically multicellular in nature and they are of various phyla, classes and families. Plants exist as flowering and no flowering in which they exhibit sexual and asexual modes of reproduction.

5. Kingdom animalia: this kingdom comprises of the more familiar green plants. They are multicellular and heterotrophic obtaining food from the bodies of plants and other animals.
   The animal kingdom can be considered as the most abundant and diverse one in comparison to the rest of the kingdoms (Wikipedia).

The definition of biodiversity mainly concentrates on the differences in species or their heterogeneity more than on the factors on to which these variables are culminate. The difference or variables in biodiversity are basically addressed at these three hierarchies; genes, species and eco-systems.

These components of biodiversity can be illustrated in figure 1 below

Figure1: Table showing examples of biodiversity components, composition and attributes

Component unit	Composition	Structure	Function
Eco-system	Ecosystems in an area	Patch size	Connectivity
Species	Species richness in area	Abundance	Predator/ prey Dynamics.
Genetic	Number of unique in an In ecological community	The relative abundance of each Unique gene in a population.	adaptation

Source: Library and Archives Canada Cataloguing in Publication Data, Main entry under title: Ecological concepts, principles and applications to conservation (2008)

Species diversity

From biology it is asserted that the species is the group of closely interrelated organisms that are capable interbreeding and resulting into fertile offspring's. In taxonomy therefore, it can be regarded as a basic unit of classification.

Species are a complete, self-generating, unique ensemble of genetic variation, capable of interbreeding and producing fertile offspring. They (and their subspecies and populations) are generally considered as the only self-replicating units of genetic diversity that can function independently (UNCED).

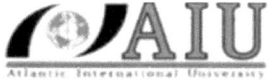
Species richness aims at estimating the number of the different species living or sharing the same habitat and where each one contributes value or an effect.

Genetic diversity

This form of biodiversity is illustrated by the genetic composition of the differing organisms but of the same species. The gene pool of the same species organisms is very narrow even when they are distant from each other. Genetic composition of an organism is not altered or determined by the environmental factors but instead it is a hereditary orientation passed on or inherited from the parent individual to the new offspring.

Determination of biodiversity can pose a challenging factor due to the fact that genes differ in dominance and hence their expression may betray the results. Some genes are dominant in which case they suppress the effect of the other they co-exist with hence on the phenotypic scale the recessive gene is marginalized or completely absent though this does not mean that it is absent in the genotype.

However, since all the observable characteristics and functionalities of organisms are renderings or derive their originality from their genetic composition, the genetic factor can be of significance in the estimation of biodiversity.

Eco-systems

These can simply be defined as self-sustainable units of the environment in which organisms of various species interact with each other. The eco-systems vary from one type to another depending on the place of location and the types of organisms occupying. However, it should be noted that some organisms are not restricted to a single type of eco-system while others are, and this characteristic is more dependant on its nature and flexibility to nature.

Take for instance the fish, whose features and behavioral activities are basically adapted to aquatic environments, and hence due to lack of environmental flexibility, it won't be able to survive the terrestrial conditions as provided by the unfavorable environment.

The significance of biodiversity to human existence

Biodiversity to man is an immediate environment from which basics of human nourishment are obtained and at the same time a great determinant in the human health and wellness. Therefore the best way to understand the effect of the environmental to human life is to establish the parameters or the underlying features on which human life connects with the immediate environment.

Ecology establishes the existence of food relationships between organisms among which are also humans because they part of the eco-system, such as the food webs and food chain. In a food

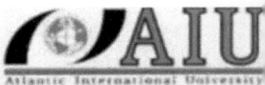
chain you will find the single direction of energy flow through eating and being eaten. While in the food web, an organism has alternative food sources varying from vegetation to animals and in all this case man exists at the most dominant position.

Another way of interluctions is through the natural habitats of forest, deserts, semi-arid and other orientations. Man can stay alone but this rendering is ineffective and short formed as we can realize with time and on considerations of our daily ventures that existence is far different from residence. Existence is supported by various factors ranging from both biotic and abiotic terms, in which case man finds great reliance on these two factors as rendered by the environment. These living organisms sharing the habitat or the immediate environment with man are of great impact to human health either positively or negatively. Discussing the disease distribution and vectors, bacteria and arthropods are always in the fore front of science study though these at the same time act as contributors for wellness and in one or the other help in advancing the adaptation to disease and medicine.

From the analysis on the human environment it is very important to conceptualize some of the underlying fundamentals in the man's existence in relation to biodiversity and this can be summed up in the following ideas;

First and fore most, the impact of man's activities in the environment is of great effect in promoting the changes on the physical world in comparison to the extent of impacts induced by the rest of the biodiversity. Consider for instance the impacts of industrialization, human settlements which have also been the dominant activities through which extinction of life has been caused in the environment due to their innovative approach which basically rotates on eliminating natural life and replacing it with modern structures.

If it is taken into consideration, assessing the effects of these activities in comparison to the effects caused by the wildlife even in the contained establishment the results will be shocking. As it will show that almost 80% of the natural life systems and food chains have been eliminated though in the wildlife containment such a percentage is impossible to be graduated. Biodiversity uses relies on items like forests and water bodies for its nourishment and yet these are the endangered or most haunted facilities of the environment by man in his venture for industrialization and settlement.

Secondly, biodiversity plays a very great epidemiological role in the distribution of disease and health in the human environment and this trend depends on the exploitation and maintenance induced onto it by man. It is evident that the majority of the pandemic outbreaks have always been spread or introduced by animal species that and that man only acts as a secondary stage in the spread cycle. The center for disease control has over the years illustrated disease prevalence and spread as originating from wildlife other than from home. This therefore, implies that disease

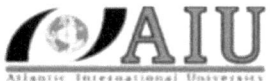
control and health wellness can also be improved and achieved through maintaining a stable immediate environment as relating to biodiversity.

Another fact to conceptualize is that the environmental biodiversity derives less material resources from man than what it contributes to man. Man is of great resource to biodiversity through social and non-material impacts and these greatly support life in the wildlife. This is applicable simply because naturally the environment can mechanize self-existence even without addition of materials or nutrients from activities; this implies that the environmental regulations and policies for maintenance are of more value than the former factor. For through policies and regulations the environment is protected from the extinctive effects of industrialization and human settlements.

In other words, it is applicable to state that the interrelationship between man and the immediate biodiversity is of more manipulative effects against the non-human organisms while favoring the human side. This should not however, be a point of celebration and pride to operate since it indicates the vulnerability of human towards extinction other than existence and this derives its fundamental fact from the supportive feature of the immediate environment. Neglecting the policies and regulations that aim to protect the environment and failure to maintaining it only cuts the branches of support that man stands on to flourish in existence and development.

The abiotic factors of the environment also play an important role in the existence of man because these enhance conditions that nourish nutrient substances used by man. The abiotic factors of the environment include; climate factor, temperatures, soil nature, PH, concentration of the air in the atmosphere.

The human environment is mainly made up of nutrient formation cycles, nutrient recycling cycles and human and environment interluctions cycles. Take for instance the carbon cycle that illustrates the value and impacts of carbon and its compounds to the human environments. According to the unified theory of ecology as stipulated by Stephen Hubbell, ecological community of sympatric species that are capable of competing in a local area for the same or similar resources, complex ecological interactions are applicable among these kind of individuals.

In other words from the unified theory it can be asserted that the differences in the structure and species orientations of individual organisms of the same ecological community exerts no implicative threat to co-existence but on the other side it only results in either competitiveness and instructiveness of the organisms. However, even under the guise of this null theory on ecological instructiveness we discover that man's activities are a great change in the game of neutrality as they culminate into negative impacts to the threat of species extinction. Therefore, instead of individual success for the various species, the human involvements or activities aggressively change the trend to demoting the success of these different individual organisms in

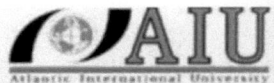
an ecological community in which asymmetric phenomena or interrelationships are introduced such as parasitism, and predation. Unfortunately these behavioral or survival orientations within the environment are not limited to non-human species but to humans niches also and calling off such a trend can be very challenging because it graviously distorts the natural equilibrium of species saturation and abundance.

What then can we say to this trend? Factually, in particular point of view you should appreciate my assertion that depicts man as the sole cause of neutrality and its distortion in the ecological community. According to the neutrality theory, all species are regarded as equivalent at a given trophic level within a food web or food chain. Hence, regardless of the environment and in this case they are equal in the parameters of; death rates, birth rates, dispersal and colonialism rates, speciation rates and in all these parameters, the different species organism will scale equally on a per-capita basis. However introducing the artificial cause of man's activities whose demands of industrialization and settlement establishments are not provided for, the extraction of row materials to support these ventures cause a great degree of entropy or instability in the ecological setup.

Perhaps it might look conflicting, that blaming man's activities is irrelevant in this case. In addition, asserting that even in natural systems there are reasonable constraints on the physical factors that can be supportive to a particular number of organisms. However, it is quite evident that though capacity has a role to play in the existence of stable biodiversity it remains premature to be the principle factor that has caused great degradation of the environment.

Chapter Two

Environmental Impacts on the Eco-Systems

The status of the natural environment stands on an equivocal point that the international community considers it a challenge against all the social and economic developments of man. The level and degree of entropy is extremely beyond measurable trends for factors that are seemingly would be underlying features for its existence, productivity, supportive or the carrying capacity and flexibility.

Science has it that naturally, the environment is supposed to be self-sustaining regardless of the influx of new Individuals and this is so because they have no gradual effect that destabilize the initial physical factors or abiotic factors onto which life relied before. As stated before that the diversity of the environment depends on the number and nature of the eco-systems contained there within so therefore on analyzing the eco-systems it is quite clear and demanding that

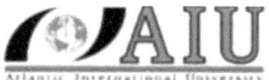
factors that are responsible for cause and distortion of eco-equilibrium are first considered key in this undertaking.

Through the various regional governments around the globe environmentalists have argued and advocated for environmental protection posing it as a mandate to the government which should may be handled through policy making and regulation forgetting that the main enemy and fore runner in the degradation of the natural environment is not the government as a body but rather the population. Possibly asserting it that this (effect of the population) still should be blamed on the government could suffice at one point may be if it is considered as the organ responsible for enforcing regulation within the population does not cover all the answers to the problems that target the environment.

Acceptably the governments have a big role and obligation to play in the minimizing of threats targeting the natural environment not through direct means but also through indirect approaches and mechanisms. The direct methods can involve the regulations, strategic policies for environment protection and maintenance, law enforcement and quarantine. These direct approaches touch the core cause and effects that the government its self has no link or connection with but they those done under the guardianship and supervision of individuals of the community for instance;

- Human settlements in wetlands; such activities are carried out by persons who in the guise of homelessness see the opportunity of free wetlands and encroaching on them even without permission or directives of the governing body. Individuals regard such areas as free provisions for the establishment of human facilities such as plantations, and homes of residence thereby cutting down all the covering vegetation and filling the wet pockets with dry land and marum for stable foundations. The value and importance of the wetlands is to filter wastes resulting from both household and industrial processes though they more so act as water pockets or reservoirs in which excess water is contained other than flooding into residence.
- Bush burning or deforestation; in most cases the sparsely populated areas are haunted by such activities where the products of tree cutting are used in timber trading and charcoal burning for instance in sub-Saharan Africa. Now charcoal is more preferred as a domestic fuel in cooking due to its smokeless feature that can allow it to be used indoors which is not a case with the firewood. Individual survey apparently indicates that non-informed persons always carry out this activity away from the eye of the environmental statutory organs of the government or even elites that know it well that deforestation is an activity that aggressively promote the extinction of habitats and the whole ecosystems.
- Degrading farming activity; under this activity we can consider the usage of chemical manure and fertilizers whose disadvantages outweighs their advantage on the soil and the product of yield, poor and unfriendly grazing methods such as zero grazing, mixed farming

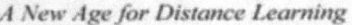

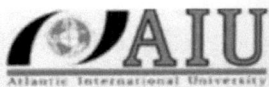

etc. Individuals concentrating on agriculture have realized the need of bulky yield from agribusiness as the only way to maximize profits due to poor pay for agricultural products most especially in the African countries. Therefore, in the pursuit to obtain huge yields they have turned on the use of chemicals under the guise of fertilizers and manure which on the other side only deprive the soil of its natural nutrient content and leave it infertile for plant production.

- House waste disposal; in so many cases, individuals have not yet realized the effect of irresponsible disposal of the common household wastes in the environment. There are little or completely no considerable parameters followed by homesteads categorizing the type of waste to be quarantined and that, which is less risky to the environment. Not necessarily, that all household waste is implicative to the environment but they vary on the compositing and the methods their recycling processes. Those wastes that are easily recyclable by the physical factors of the environment and soil can be considered to be less implicative however some material such as the packing bags made from plastic and poly-ethene are very dangerous, posing threats of life extinction for the soil animals.

On the other hand, however, the indirect approach concentrates on the facilities, which have the government patent clearing them to proceed with their activities where some of which are environmental hazards. In so many cases, the governments have granted permission of operation to some multinational companies even without considering or evaluating their environmental impacts and the implications of such impacts to human health and general life status of the ecosystems. The indirect phenomenon is that the government on one point think is rendering services to the public such as employment and good infrastructure but yet the hazards imbedded in these vast establishments are life threatening.

The resulting effect is that such establishments are even protected by the government that may be doing it under the guise of promoting development and boosting the job market at a national level for its citizens. Take for instance the impacts of industrialization on the environment as they can be categorized into positive and negative patterns.

For the purposes of the environment assessment perhaps we can consider pollution which is also negative impact to the environment as resulting from industrialization. The polluter substances from automobiles and the stationary plantations, consumables have nothing good that they add to the environment but only destroying the environment by attacking the three basic parameters of biodiversity; species, genetic and ecosystems respectively.

The effect of pollution propagates in a stepwise trend starting from the smallest unit of biodiversity, the gene. As illustrated in the schematic flow cycle (figure. 2) below, the effect of the pollutant bulges remarkably as it transcends from one level to the next one within the environment.

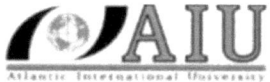

Notwithstanding its absorptive capacity by the environment that also increases gradually such that by the period it ramifies to the top hierarchy in the environment, which is the ecosystem its concentration in the biotic factors of the environment is corrosive and detrimental to all forms of life that make up the complete ecosystem.

Figure 2: Stepwise Propagative Circulation of the Pollutant in the Environmental Levels

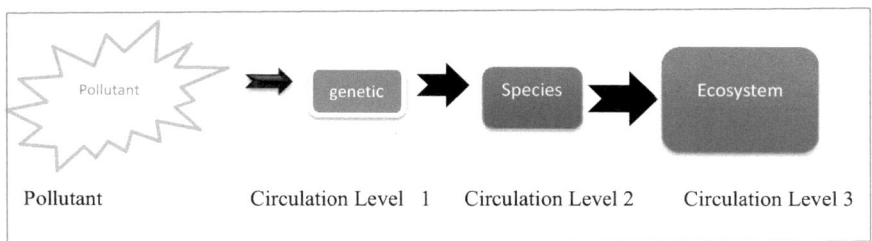

At the Genetic Level

All pollutants are chemically contaminative to the biochemistry of the natural living systems of both plants and animals to the extent that some these substances can alter the normal functioning of the cells. However, pollutants can cause alterations only when they are directly attacking the nucleus that controls the cellular activities which also contains the genetic or hereditary material for both prokaryotic and eukaryotic cells.

The effect of the polluting chemical also vary from one individual to another as organisms differ in genetic composition it may not affect all individuals in the same trend or the effect to some individuals its impact may depend on the levels of concentration taken into the body. the absorptive capacity which is the quantity of pollutant that the environment can take in at each of these levels also depends on a number of factors varying from composition of the pollutant, percentages concentrations of the substance constituents, medium of disposal (water, or air) etc.

Secondly, the effect of the pollutant at the genetic level is of less impact to the environment as compared in the other levels because ecological niche of the genes is only internal within the body hence even within the same habitat other organs may take long to contract the effects as obtained by the primary recipient.

The Species Level

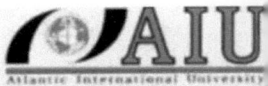
The pollutants at the species level has already managed to circulate the entire transport channels of the organism and then it's effects can be channeled to other individuals of the same species in the closest range of the habitat. Assuming that all the physical or abiotic factors of the environment are kept constant, substances of contamination have suitable species of individuals within the family where the acceleration of their absorptive capacity is gradual as compared to others.

The species level is of great value within the construction and structuring of ecosystems that are made from food webs and food chains in which the trophic levels are represented by species organisms. Therefore, the circulation capacity of the chemical is of great impact towards the environment as compared to that in the first level.

The Ecosystem Level

All individuals within the environment forming food webs and food chains build and support the ecosystems.

Within food chains, chemicals or pollutants accumulate at each succeeding trophic level until they reach the quaternary consumers or scavengers' and at this point, their concentration is fatal or lethal to some extent in the living system. Take for example the DDT chemical used in the prevention of malaria spread by mosquitoes most especially in the third world countries. The substance is mainly targeting the distortion of mosquito reproductive cycles though the end results are more pervasive to all living systems even of those who are supposedly aimed to be protected. The introduction of DDT at the initial cycles of the mosquito larvae stages enrolls the chemical into the ecosystem as these are eaten by small birds and other organisms in the aquatic habitat. However the chemical is also absorbed through inhalation directly from air by humans in which case the concentrations are less as compared to those taken in through indirect means for example in the interactions within the food webs and food chains.

Within an ecological community, it should be noted that at each successive feeding or trophic level the size of the feeding individual increases. Though this may not commonly or necessarily mean increased food consumption, however this increased body volume relatively acquire a higher volume of the circulation or transport medium such as the blood and the tissue fluid and in this case also the concentration of the absorbed pollutant is increased.

An ecological survey carried out by the National Environmental Management Authority (NEMA) to determine the trends of the DDT accumulation in the human environments showed a cumulative pattern for with each successive year of data collections. The data samples collected from the circulation systems of common domestic animals and the results below were obtained (figure 3).

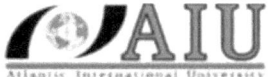
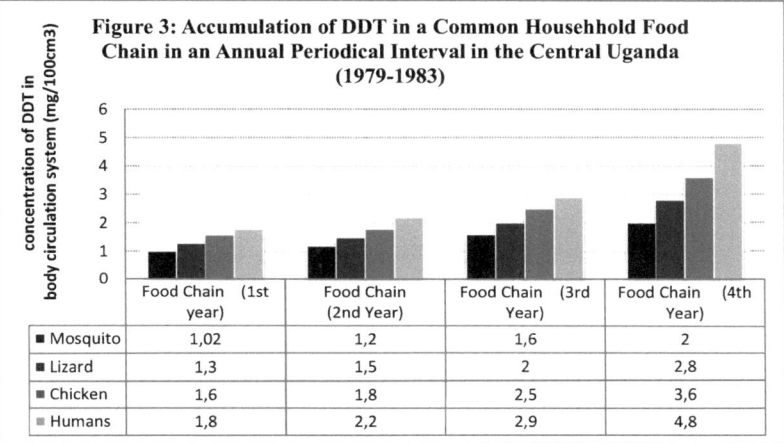

Figure 3: Accumulation of DDT in a Common Household Food Chain in an Annual Periodical Interval in the Central Uganda (1979-1983)

concentration of DDT in body circulation system (mg/100cm3)

	Food Chain (1st year)	Food Chain (2nd Year)	Food Chain (3rd Year)	Food Chain (4th Year)
■ Mosquito	1,02	1,2	1,6	2
■ Lizard	1,3	1,5	2	2,8
■ Chicken	1,6	1,8	2,5	3,6
■ Humans	1,8	2,2	2,9	4,8

Adapted from the National Environment Management Authority (NEMA) archives for DDT circulation trends human domestic environments (1985)

Chapter Three

Principles and Fundamentals in Environmental Impact Assessment

Descriptively, the phrase environmental impact assessment can be explained as the process that involves the identification, prediction, evaluation and the mitigation of the biophysical, social and other related effects of development proposals prior to major decisions being taken and commitments made with the aim of environmental sustainability (IAIA). This activity not only aim at finding out the state of the environment but it goes further to give strategies and approaches through which the pending matters on the scaling of environmental equilibrium are to be balanced.

in the pursuit to assess the impact of the environment the key targets aimed include the determination of ecological community of the environment which vary from marine to terrestrial ecosystems, the productivity of the environment due to its biodiversity, the threatening risks and their source, and so many other factors can be put under this consideration.

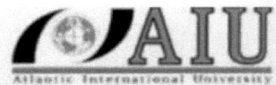
The origin of this process has its root from international bodies and association of environmentalists fore ran by the International Association for Impact Assessment (IAIA) and the Institute Of Environmental Assessment, UK (IEA). These also saw the importance in evaluating human impacts on the natural environment as a fundamental pillar in designing schemes and projects through which the environment can be protected and increase its productivity. Currently in the international point of view, the majority of the regional states have legislated the policy of impact assessment such as the United States, Portugal, England, and other European countries.

J. Holder stated, "EIAs are unique in that they do not require adherence to a predetermined environmental outcome, but rather they require decision -makers to account for environmental values in their decisions and to justify those decisions in light of detailed environmental studies and public comments on the potential environmental impacts of the proposal". In other words the results of the findings collected by the environmental impact assessment organs (EIA's) is then presented to the environmental technocrats for easy planning and strategizing through human projects where environmental risks results from and use these as the very channels in enforcing and implementing reliable projects for the environment.

However, is needful for good results of this study venture to ascertain and identify the desired key points of the environment under the pressure of pervasive human projects and this can start by outlining the existing and possible ecosystems in the nearest vicinity. Ecosystems are the targets of almost every environmental hazard and it will be a waste of time and resources to embark on assessing the impact of the environment without considering the biodiversity of the ecological community. In the table below the most important ecosystems have been listed with their respective subdivisions according to the TEEB (The Economics of Ecosystems and Biodiversity).

Figure 4: Classification of Ecosystems Used In the Economics of Ecosystems and Biodiversity

No.	Main Biomes –Level 1	Subdivisions In Biomes-Ecosystems
1.	**Marine/ open ocean**	i. Open ocean ii. Coral leafs
2.	**Costal systems**	i. Sea grass/ algae beds ii. Shelf sea iii. Estuaries iv. Shores (rocky and beaches)
3.	**wetlands**	Coastal wetlands i. Tidal marsh ii. Mangroves Inland wetlands

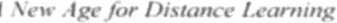
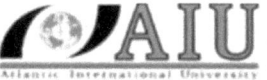
		i.	Flood plains
		ii.	Peat-wetlands (begs, fens etc.)
4.	Lakes/ rivers	i.	Lakes
		ii.	Rivers
5.	forests	Tropical forests
		i.	Tropical rain forests
		ii.	Tropical dry forests
		Temperate forests
		i.	Temperate rain/ evergreen
		ii.	Temperate deciduous forests
6.	Woodland and shrub land	i.	Heathland
		ii.	Mediterranean scrub
		iii.	Various scrubland
7.	Grass/rangeland	i.	Savanna
8.	Desert	i.	Semi desert
		ii.	True desert (sand /rock)
9.	Tundra	i.	Tundra
10. 0	Ice/rock/polar	i.	Ice/rock/polar
11.	Cultivated	i.	Cropland (arable land, pastures, etc.)
		ii.	Plantations / orchards / agro-forestry, etc.
		iii.	Aquaculture / rice paddies, etc.
12.	Urban	i.	Urban

Source: Based on mix of classifications, mainly MA (2005a) and Costanza et al. (1997) which in turn are based on classifications from US Geol. Survey, IUCN, WWF, UNEP and FAO.

Principles in Environmental Impact Assessment

In the plan to conduct an elaborate environment impact assessment it is recommended to identify the principles to be involved and the their interconnectedness in the process. This serves the purpose of following the right sequence and pattern in achieving or a step by step methodology within this undertaking.

Two principles have been outlined in this business and these are basic and operational. The basic principles serve to meet the strategic policies, plans and programs in environmental protection. The differing feature between the basic and the operational is that the later one describes how the former one should be implemented or applied in the due process. Therefore, in simplicity it is quite applicable to assert that the basic principles are the practical tools to be used in the activity of environmental impact assessment whereas the operational principles are the wheels on to which the tools are to be carried towards their desired target. The basic principles are fixed and pose to have no room of substation though among them exist a great trend of interdependency a feature calls for a systematic approach that is unalterable.

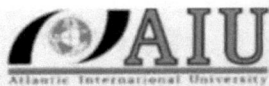
The basic principles to be followed in assessing the impact of the environment are explained in the following lines;

- ❖ **Purposive:** the process being followed should have a given number of set objectives and aims that are regarded as goals appropriate for the assessment. Effective environmental impact assessment is mainly calibrated by using its purpose notwithstanding the expected outcomes. This principle helps the technical team to stay focused while collecting data such that it only considers the relevant information in line with the purpose of the activity.

- ❖ **Rigorous:** this principle emphasizes the application of best practicable science, and the usage of methodologies and techniques appropriate to address the problems of the environment under investigation. Rigor principally demands for core practical and applicable techniques in the assessment process and its main purpose is to leave no room for inaccurate and inconsistent data.

- ❖ **Practical:** the process should emphasize the practical knowledge based extraction and collection that can be helpful in problem solving. The practical approach allows easiness and flexibility of the process such that it is also acceptable and easily implementable by proponents.

- ❖ **Relevant:** The environment is a wide topic on to which you should expect contributions from different sources. This therefore, calls for ascertaining the quality of data and its relevancy to the process undertaken in assessing the environmental impact.

- ❖ **Cost-effective:** while designing the process to be followed in the assessment venture of the environmental impact it should be noted that the resources available have a limit. Otherwise if there is no considerable limitations within the time, available information, and methodology it may pose a great challenge in achieving the intended goals of the process.

- ❖ **Efficiency:** Though it is not wise to be spend-shrift in joint ventures in order to prevent loss of focus and endangering future analysis, but yet this does not necessarily call for inadequacy of resources. To prevent weariness and anxiety within the team the adequate resources should be provided to achieve efficiency and effectiveness and these will still range from cost of burdens in terms of time and finance.

- ❖ **Focused:** The intention under this principle is to be sure that the results from the assessment will remarkably be helpful in designing strategies and policies that support the productivity and sustainability of the environment. Staying focused can pose a serious challenge most especially when it comes to joint ventures however, to minimize these sort of

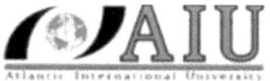

diversions areas of weaknesses should be analyzed as early as possible in the orientation phase.

❖ **Adaptive:** the proposal life cycle should be attractive to all possible sources of data and to the team member's opinion. This helps to eliminate any practice of monopoly that might corrupt and marginalize the findings in which case they will be imbalanced.

❖ **Participative:** the process under proposal should encourage the intake and participation of the interested public with relevant ideas and aims to the proposal of the project. The benefit resulting from this principle is that the decision making team is provided with multiple ideas, data, intellectual expertise and knowledge which it uses in achieving the intended goals easily.

❖ **Interdisciplinary:** Bernice Goldsmith et al. states that such a process should ensure that the appropriate techniques and experts in the relevant biophysical and socio-economic disciplines are employed, including use of traditional knowledge as relevant.

❖ **Credible:** the assessment process is considered to be an activity aiming at finding facts and not fictions and for this reason therefore, professionalism, rigor, fairness, objectivity, impartiality, and balance plus the need to be subject towards the independent checks and verifications.

❖ **Integrated:** all credible environment impact assessment processes should show great interrelationships of social, economic and biophysical aspects. Since this is to be handled in form of a research it is advisable to reference and borrow ideas and facts from the various spheres of human involvements.

❖ **Transparent:** the environment is a facility freely enjoyed and manipulated by all humans and therefore, the need to be outspoken is of great value for credulity of the assessment process. The public should therefore have free access to the results of each phase in the due process.

❖ **systematic:** according to the analysis as explained by Bernice Goldsmith et al. this assessment process should result in full consideration of all relevant information on the affected environment, of proposed alternatives and their impacts, and of the measures necessary to monitor and investigate residual effects.

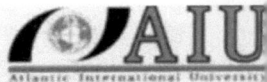
The operational principles

These principle act as the driving wheels onto which the basic principles fuel the proposal or process life cycle however, their importance or significance may not be achieved appropriately if they are not applied as early as possible.

Also important in this criterion is that these operational principles should be in internationally agreed measures and activities otherwise there strength and weaknesses depend a lot on their interdependence on the already revised and recommended assessment parameters at an international scale. These principles include;

1. screening
2. scoping
3. examination of alternatives
4. impact analysis
5. mitigation and impact management
6. evaluation of significance
7. preparation of environmental impact statement or report
8. review of the environment impact statement (EIS)
9. decision making
10. Follow up.

The main stepwise operational principles have been conceptionalized in framework scheme that can be followed while carrying out the assessment plan.

However, before implementation of the operational principles it is recommendable to analyse topics in this venture, and also determining the trends involved. The Australian environmental protection for the marine biodiversity has progressively designed a framework of strategies to be taken into consideration while embarking on the assessment of the environmental impact most especially when the objectives are concentrating on the protection and conservation of the marine biodiversity. For even when the research is mainly at assessing, it is important to carry out a systematic evaluation through the process that is to be used and this activity helps in identifying the subject of the survey, the duration and the resources to be used in the process.

Technically this is one way of planning for the assessment program or project and it considers a lot of factors, and questions as well as analyzing a great number of strategies proposed so that the best concepts are adapted for the best results. This will require prioritizing of the assessment as the capstone in restoring the natural equilibrium of the environment before anything else is done to help the threatening issues.

The risks threatening the environment can be assessed following the evaluation framework designed by the marine biodiversity environmental protection unit (figure5).

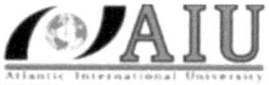
**Figure 5: Proposed Framework in the Evaluation of the Process Used In Risk Assessment
of the Marine Biodiversity in Australia**

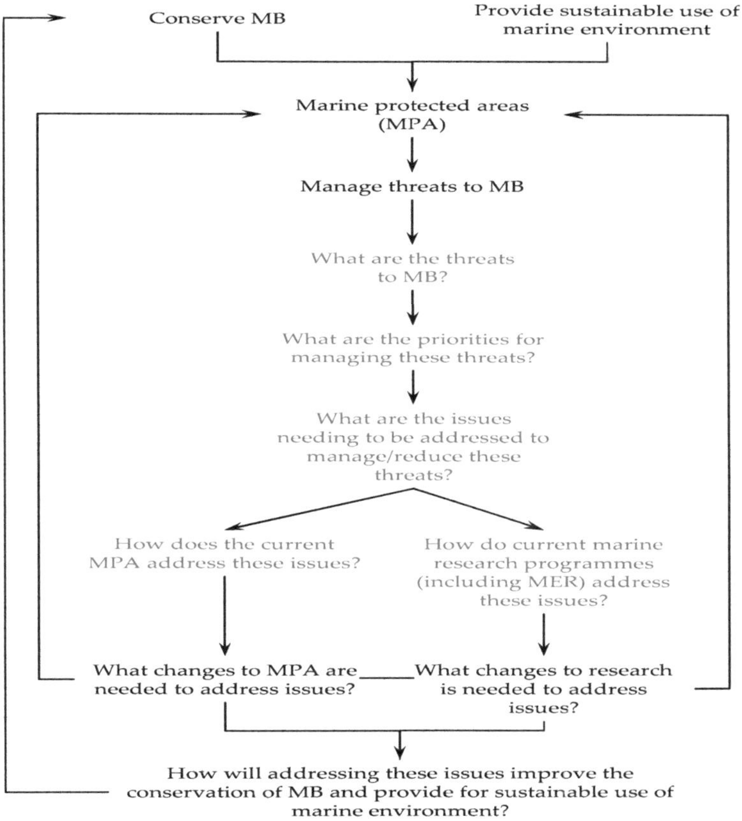

Conserve MB   Provide sustainable use of
marine environment

Marine protected areas
(MPA)

Manage threats to MB

What are the threats
to MB?

What are the priorities for
managing these threats?

What are the issues
needing to be addressed to
manage/reduce these
threats?

How does the current
MPA address these issues?   How do current marine
research programmes
(including MER) address
these issues?

What changes to MPA are
needed to address issues?   What changes to research
is needed to address
issues?

How will addressing these issues improve the
conservation of MB and provide for sustainable use of
marine environment?

Source: R16;A briefing/update/overview of the DPI Karen Astles risk assessment project
regarding threats from human induced disturbances, including projected timeframes. (2008)

This evaluation framework is both pre and post methodological application in the assessment
process i.e. it addresses the factors to be considered before starting the evaluation process and at
the same time it is used to answer the question that would arise from the process when finished.
Though the framework is conceptual and designed for assessing the risks facing a marine

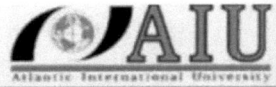
ecosystem there will be little or negligible differences when applied to the environmental assessment of other common ecosystems.

Model of principle application

As remarked earlier, that the operational principles work in a stepwise approach and there exist a pattern of interdependency among them and therefore there should a revised systematic cycle to follow while applying them. Just like any human living system that would find operational difficulty if the internal environment is not in equilibrium so it the case with these principles.

For better analysis and understanding of these concepts and fundamentals used in the environmental impact assessment, we can borrow ideas elaborated by Achieng Ogola.

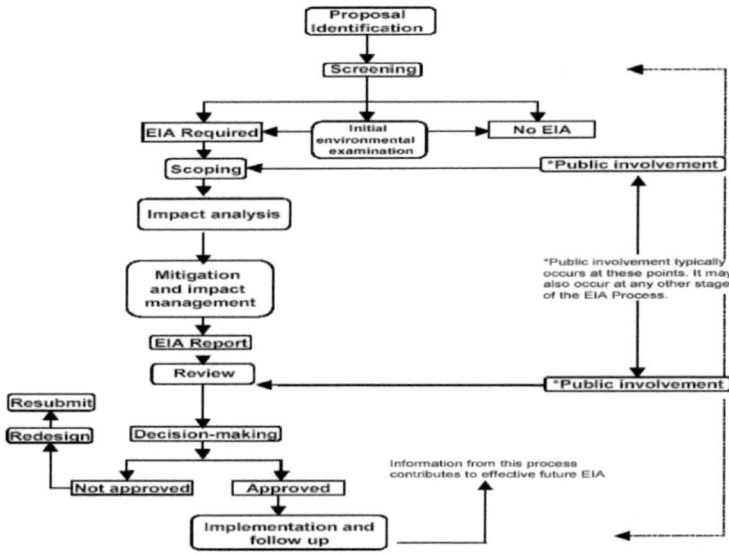

Figure 5: Presented at Short Course II on Surface Exploration for Geothermal Resources, organized by UNU-GTP and KenGen, at Lake Naivasha, Kenya, 2-17 November 2007

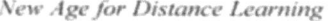
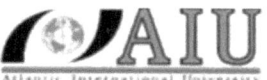

The screening activity: the main objective aimed at in screening is to determine or to establish the proposal is relevant and can be subjected to the environmental impact assessment. Screening also determines the level of detail offered by the subject and at this stage, it can be asserted that the filtration or sieving of parameters is carried out considerably.

The scoping stage: this stage serves to identify and mark out the key issues and impacts that are possibly acceptable or of great importance while establishing the terms of reference for an efficient environmental impact assessment plan. The activity of scoping in this assessment process is

(a). for the identification of important issues that are to be concentrated on while handling an environmental assessment project. These issues comprise of the baseline and the alternatives.

(b). to determine the appropriate time interval and lifelong boundaries to be allocated for the assessment of the environment.

(c). To determine the source of reliable information that is necessary in the process of decision-making.

(d). Also to anticipate the significant effects and factors to be studied in details.

The assessment stage: this undertaking can involve both the examination of the alternatives and impact analysis. These are key holders for establishing the preferred or environmentally remarkable and benign option for out sourcing the proposal objectives and at the same time the later helps in the identification and prediction of the likely environmental, social and other related effects arising from the proposal.

Reviewing of the process: this practice centralizes on the designing the environmental impact statement which is the element of the review stage. The statement or report documentizes clearly the impacts of the proposal. The report also serves to elaborate the significance of the effects and the concerns of the curious audience arising from the general public and perhaps the related communities as touched by the proposal.

The environmental impact statement (report)

This is the final report produced by the functional team showing the outcomes of the environmental assessment process. The content and structure of this statement have always been determined by national however, some multilateral and bilateral organisations who are stake holders in environmental management have also played a contribution to this design. This means therefore, the structure of the environmental assessment report will considerably vary from one state to another as dependant on the national laws and policies of a particular regional state in conjunction with the related organs beside the government.

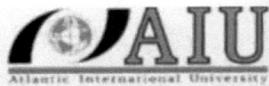
Though changes and differences cannot be eliminated, the following details are important to be included in the assessment report;

1. An executive summary;-introduces the introductory prehumble.
2. Policy, legal and administrative framework;- shows the hierarchy of the authoritative and commissioning body.
3. The description of the environment;- shows the ecosystem under scrutiny.
4. Description of the proposed project in detail;- elaborates the components and processes to be involved.
5. Significant environmental impacts;-outlines of the key impacts to be checked or targets of the assessment.
6. Socio-economic analysis of project impacts;- indicates the implications of the proposed project in the social and economic arenas of human involvements.
7. Identifications and analysis of alternatives;- outlines the other possible approaches through which the assessment can be rendered.
8. The mitigation action or the intended mitigation management plan;- illustrates the revised procedures that tend to minimize the critical patterns in the process.
9. Environmental management plan;- proposes the revised mechanism through which the environment can be maintained and protected from the common threats.
10. Monitoring program;- shows the proposed schedules, schemes and methods to be used in the follow up process.
11. Knowledge gaps;- shows the pending parts of the review or project where knowledge and information content can be adjusted.
12. The public involvement;- this part shows the pattern, capacity and the roles of the public in the assessment process.
13. List of references;- this part can act as the bibliography showing the sources of knowledge and information applied in the assessment process.
14. The chapter of appendices;- it is expected for the report to include some extracts of environmental scenes, diagrams and frameworks. All these are contained in the appendices chapter.

Decision-making: this level takes the determing factors into consideration and finalize the importance of the assessment before the strategies are implemented while using the outcomes of the assessment.

The implementation stage: the outcomes of the assessment proposal we assume that at this level they have been materialized and ready for usage. The implementation stage serves to use these results of the assessment in devising methods and strategies that will achieve the positive results onto which the environment is to be handled.

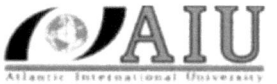
Monitoring/Audit (follow up): According to the analysis as stipulated by the IAIA, the follow up stage ensures that the terms and condition of approval are met; to monitor also impacts the development and the effectiveness of mitigation measures. In addition, this strengthens future EIA applications and mitigation measures; and, where required, to undertake environmental audit and process evaluation to optimize environmental management. It is desirable, whenever possible, if monitoring, evaluation and management plan indicators are designed so they also contribute to local, national and global monitoring of the state of the environment and sustainable development (IAIA).

Chapter Four

Policy Implications and the Institutional Framework in EIA

As noted earlier, the policy trends are nation dependant and therefore, they are not on an international pass mark since each nation's sovereignty is to be preserved. However, this does not rule out the role of international bodies   that pursue environmental protection and maintenance.

In a global perspective, it can realized that the idea of environmental impact assessment has not yet been totally embraced by all the world society for the reasons of it being anew ideology and at the same time the concepts unexplained properly.

First of all, this new trend in achieving environmental stability and biodiversity protection has showed with challenging approaches where it poses threats to individuals who have not been under scrutiny in their exploitation of the environment. These are not only individuals but also multi-personal organisations and businesses which have predated on the biodiversity of our common ecosystem under the cover of poorly revised policies that don't check their activities. It is such systems and organisations that embarrasses the strategies in EIA's.

Secondly, EIA's activities are not the threat implicating the activities of individuals but rather what is the outcomes of the assessment going to be used and how this affect the environment and those that depend on it. These questions are the source of all the legal and policy dynamics that are induced by environmental impact assessment. For instance if at the stage of impact analysis in the project process the rising issue is the impact of pollution out running for the industries and factories within the environment such as those that empty their wastes into the aquatic environment.

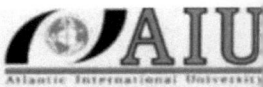
What should these companies expect after the assessment is evident that their activities are to be compromised if not terminated but because these are the source of good and huge revenue for the government to support such projects there will be a jolt in the structuring of regulations and at the same time, the policies will be fettered.

Therefore, due to such reasons and considerations the EIA process is still shackled and infirmitized in the regional governments which is an issue that calls for attention of multinational bodies that operate with global statutes. Basically the key nations in the environmental impact assessment movement are Australia, England, Canada and the USA. In these countries, the environmental impact assessment policies have been imbedded and installed into the state laws and regulations that advocate and protect the activities of the EIA projects.

The financial support and legal protection have been provided to such projects as a way to promote the transparency and public involvement in the practice. The legal and policies related to the activities of EIA projects have been supported legally by the follow up process which is mainly carried out under the observation and supervision of the statutory organs of the government alongside the environment technical team.

These regional states that are key in promoting the environmental impact assessment programs have taken up the role of revising the environment assessment statements or reports checking up where the strategies in management of the environment should be applied and the key targets of the screening and scoping process. The main role of the report is not to document the outcomes of the assessment by it is used by the enforcement teams of the government and international organisations to plan by averting the dreaded threats that the assessed impacts are posing or inducing onto the environment.

Therefore the assessment report is key in the process of structuring and designing policies by the legal bodies of the regional governments and this according to my opinion can help us to track the policies and their trends from one state to another.

Hence, after this concept it is coherent to assert that in the place where the environmental assessment report not been laid out or produced little or completely no strategy has been structured by the state to manage environmental biodiversity and the ecosystems are therefore under direct vulnerability for distortion and final extinction.

International Environmental Law Context and the Environmental Impact Assessment

(a) Espoo 1991

This is a trans-boundary convention which addressed the environmental impact assessment programs at a multilateral pattern. It was the first of this kind and it mainly proposes or stipulates the involved parties and their roles during the assessment process. The treaty lays out the obligations of the multiple parties involved and that of the involved states such that

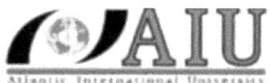
awareness is raised for each individual state to demarcate the projects under assessment in these criteria.

The Espoo convention does not stop at only stipulating the roles and responsibilities of the multiple states involved and the related parties but it goes on also to elaborates or provide provisions for principle and procedures to be followed and the list of activities, contents and documents that are involved in this criterion.

(b) The Rio declaration (1992)

The convention that progressed in 1992 established an article (17) that stipulates the function of Environmental Impact Assessment. The Rio declaration on environment and development emphasizes the use of the EIA and its outcomes in states as a tool to be applied in strategizing the plans intended for national development such as in the construction of infrastructures in the regional states. Also the principle 15 of the declaration considers EIA as a precautionary approach in principle implementation states Acieng Ogola.

The Rio declaration agenda 21 which also acted as the result of the convention rendered the following obligations to the regional governments;

❖ *That they emphasize the "Promotion for the development of appropriate methodologies for making integrated energy, environment and economic policy decisions for sustainable development, inter alia, through environmental impact assessment (9.12(b))*
❖ *Implement the Development, improvement and strategically apply environmental impacts assessment, to foster sustainable industrial development (9.18)*
❖ *Carry out investment analysis and feasibility studies including environmental assessments for establishing forest based processing enterprises*
❖ *Introduce appropriate EIA procedures for proposed projects likely to have significant impacts upon biological diversity, providing for suitable information to be made widely available and for public participation, where appropriate, and encourage the assessment of impacts of relevant policies and programs on biological diversity (15.5(k)"(UNICED 1992).*

Further still, the agenda 21 goes on to improvise parameters or patterns to nations that should be observed while establishing the environmental statutes or regulations. Some of the suggested patterns are given below;

1. UN Convention on climate change and Biological Diversity (1992) cited EIA as an implementing mechanism of these conventions (article 4 and 14 respectively).
2. Doha Ministerial Declaration encourages countries to share expertise and experience with members wishing to perform environmental reviews at the national level (November 2001).

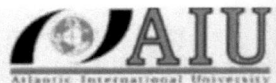
3. UNECE (Aarhus) Convention on Access to Information, Public Participation in Decision Making and Access to Justice in Environmental Matters (1998) covers the decisions at the level of projects and plans, programs and policies and by extension, applies to EIA and SEA
4. United Nations Conference on the Environment in Stockholm 1972. (UNICED 1992)

Chapter Five

Final Overview: Recommendations and Conclusion

Recommendations

The importance of the environment is universal to all humans and more surprising this applies in all spheres of man's socio-economic development parameters. The assessment program helps to update the stakeholders in environmental management plan about the loopholes in the strategies and activities that expose the environment to extensive threats. The threatening issues against the environment are categorised into the natural cause and the artificial factors.

The natural cause of threats mainly includes the natural conditions of the environment to which sometimes man has little force to alter. Take for instance the tragic hurricanes that have always claimed large numbers of innocent lives in Asia and in the American states. Such happenings and tragedies cannot be stooped but or very little alterations can be effected by man in controlling their direction and region of impact but yet is so possible for man to reduce on the impacts of such calamities on to his environment.

There is no place for excusing man while blaming the damage caused to human settlements by natural causes on to these factors themselves. This is so simply because man is the sole cause of the majority of these adverse calamities and therefore there is need for him to carry his own burden in halting the side effects of his activities that could be causing directly or indirectly contributing to the abrupt existence of these environmental calamities. For instance the problem of global warming which is currently taking the front seat among the global threats that are questioning the destiny and remaining life span of human existence.

While considering the possible ways of altering these natural calamities, it might certainly pose to be a chase of the air. This is because they are nature hence altering them is not in the powers of man but belongs to the more sovereign and supreme entity however, as noted in the previous lines that man can only reduce on their effects is acceptable and hence his next plan should be devising the strategies that can achieve this. Such strategies can range from installation of technological systems in different global locations that predict the calamity before their existence such human settlements are also strategically located where they won't be aggressively attacked.

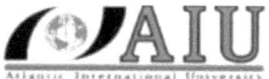
However, for the artificial causes there seem to be need for the regional governments to come to terms through treaties and revise policies and regulations that can change the sequence of the threats.

The recent Davos world convention that concentrated on the solutions to control and avert the effects posed by global warming showed the ability of achieving world stability and environmental safety among nations. Regardless of the political differences among the nations it was agreed on that the first step should be obligations played by the regional states in cutting the carbon dioxide emissions and increasing the green covering with in their respective regions and environments.

Therefore, international conventions and multilateral treaties are great game changers most especially when it comes to averting global threats.

Conclusion

Briefly, instead of limiting the environmental management to statutory bodies it will be of great benefit if the public is openly involved in this undertaking for better strategies. The strategies have always been outlined in the regional governments and even sometimes tried but they have materialized nothing or less to environment protection.

This should be blamed on the negligence shown towards the assessment projects in other words the idea of environmental impact assessment has not been principally embraced in most of the world states or even embraced but not in the right way as recommended according to the revised approaches.

A lot has to be done in the implementation of the strategies and this should begin with individual concerns of the public, in which sense it should be among the principle aims for the government to sell the environmental management passion and idea to the local communities through friendly means that attract the transparency of the government policies.

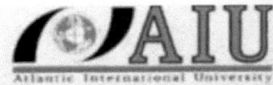
Bibliography

1. Achieng Ogola Pacifica. F: Environmental Impact Assessment General Procedures. http://www.kengen.co.gov

2. Bernice Goldsmith et al. Principles of Environmental Impact Assessment Best Practice; (1999).link at http://www.iaia.org

3. CBD-Convention on Biological Diversity, UNEP-United Nations Environment Programme, Handbook of the Convention on Biological Diversity (Earthscan Publications Ltd., London, UK, 1992)

4. Elden Enger et al.: Concepts in Biology; 12th edition (2007). Published by Mc Graw Hill high education. New York USA

5. Holder, J., (2004), Environmental Assessment: The Regulation of Decision Making, Oxford University Press, New York

6. http:// www.biodiversitybc.org: Ecological concepts, principles and applications to conservation. Canada

7. http://www.wikipedia.com: The origin of the Biological species and the animal Kingdom

8. International Authority for Impact Assessment (IAIA) and the Environmental Impact Assessment, UK: Principles of Environmental Impact Assessment Best Practice; (1999).link at http://www.iaia.org

9. M. B.V. Roberts et al: Biology, Advanced Topics 4th edition (1985). Published by the Oxford university press UK

10. P.M. Muchiri: Principles of Biology; 3rd Edition. Vol.2, (2006). Published by Pezi publishers Ltd. Nairobi Kenya

11. United Nations Conference on Environment and Development (UNCED-1992) and summarized by Bunnell, F.L. 1998. Managing forests to sustain biodiversity: substituting accomplishment for motion. Forestry Chronicle

12. UNICED 1992: UNICED Report A/CONF. 151/5/Rev 1

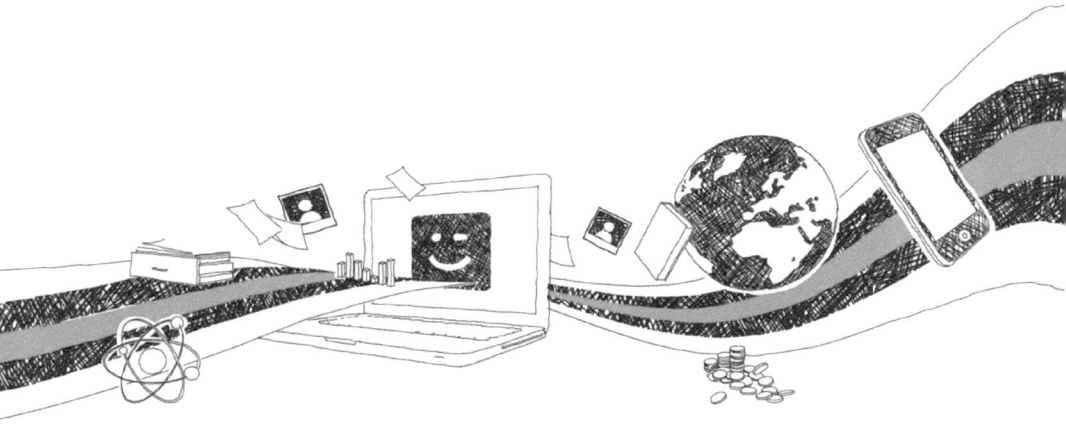
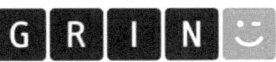